Introduction

Here at www.FunctionalLabz.com we believe you can have fun and get in great shape without costly gym memberships and without taking hours out of your day.

We're all about fun, fast, and highly effective functional workouts that help you reach your health and fitness goals without wasting your time.

This book is full of quick, intense kettlebell workouts intended to build muscle, burn fat, and improve overall fitness.

Inside you'll find…

- AMRAP's
- Rounds
- Tabata's
- EMOM's
- Timed Intervals
- and more variety to prevent boredom and keep thing interesting.

Have fun, and please feel free to reach out with any questions or feedback.

~Ryan☐

Benefits of Kettlebell Training

Though workouts can be challenging to fit into your everyday schedule, it is important to implement a daily routine that is realistic and will keep you motivated. Exercising with kettlebells is an extremely easy and convenient way to get a complete total body workout. Kettlebells are easy to incorporate into your daily workout routine because they are convenient, easy to store in any home gym and provide your body with complete overall training.

Total Body Workout - Kettlebells are great because they allow for a full body workout. They can be used for strength, weight loss, endurance, and can help with your cardio routines. They help you gain strength in all areas of your body. Whether you are a beginner or an expert, kettlebells can build stronger legs, arms, shoulders, and core muscles. They are convenient because they can be stored out of sight or can be your go-to equipment when you workout at home. Your daily workouts can be greatly enhanced by incorporating this simple piece of equipment into your regular routine.

Core Strength - The core muscles in your body provide proper balance and stability. Having strong core muscles improves your body's overall function. With strong back and abdomen muscles, we are less likely to succumb to back pain and other issues that cause people to become immobile. Strong core muscles allow for better posture and reduces strain on the spine. Kettlebells are an excellent workout tool to strengthen and improve core muscles. The kettlebells awkward weight and shape allows you to work the core muscles during almost any exercise, whether you're specifically targeting the core or not.

Improve Movement and Coordination - For athletes who are training in any particular sport, it is important to be in tip-top shape. Since most sports require athletes to be coordinated, agile, and fast, kettlebells are an excellent way for athletic individuals to increase their speed and improve performance. Exercises such as kettlebell swings, cleans, and snatches increase power and strength in the hip area which in turn increases an athlete's speed and explosiveness.

Burn Fat – Body fat can be harmful to your health and devastating to your fitness. It is important to establish a regular functional fitness routine that helps your body burn fat. A proper diet combined with an effective workout routine is a great way to control bodyweight. Working out with kettlebells is an excellent way to boost your cardio and burn unwanted calories. For beginners, a simple fat burning routine could consist of several repetitions of squats and presses. For a more advanced workout, kettlebells can be used for deadlifts, power olympic lifts, and other compound movements that work the entire body and burn fat. Either one of these workout routines will help to burn fat and build core muscles.

Cardio - Because kettlebells are so versatile, they provide individuals with strength training and allow you to burn fat while building muscle. During a regular workout routine with kettlebells, you're not only building muscle but you're increasing your cardio strength. For individuals who prefer less impact during their cardio workouts, kettlebells are a great alternative. The purpose of a cardio workout is to increase your heart rate. The compound, full-body movements involved in kettlebell workouts are an excellent way to increase heart rate and burn calories.

Lower Body Strength - Lower body strength is important in many sporting activities. What most people don't understand is lower body strength is also important for everyday function. Since the lower part of our bodies contain the largest muscle in our bodies - the gluteus maximus, it is important for this area of the body to be worked on a regular basis. Increasing lower body strength helps prevent injuries and accidental falls. Even if you are not an athlete, using kettlebells to improve lower body strength, balance, and coordination is a great way to make you more capable and functional during day-to-day activities.

Increase Flexibility and Mobility - For athletes, flexibility and mobility are critical in their performance. Functional, compound kettlebell movements can help athletes increase range of motion and improve overall performance. For non-athletes, kettlebell workouts are just as effective at improving mobility and flexibility in the joint areas. For individuals looking to become more mobile, simple kettlebell exercises can help achieve desired results.

Build Muscle - The use of kettlebells to build muscle mass is often preferred to that of barbells. Individuals who use kettlebells are more likely interested in building lean, functional muscle as opposed to bulky muscles. Adding kettlebells to your workout routine will help get you the lean muscular body you desire and allow you the ability to be mobile.

Improve Grip Strength - Another benefit to kettlebell workouts is grip strength. On the surface, this may not be as important of a factor as building core muscle or burning fat, but some workout experts beg to differ. Grip strength is essential in obstacle races and any workout that requires the use of free weights or that requires you to grip a piece of equipment. The consistent use of kettlebells during your workout can significantly improve the strength of your grip. The unique design of kettlebells provides an intense workout for your forearms, wrists and fingers. The stronger a person's grip the better their workout routine will be.

Improve Balance - The use of kettlebells can give a strong indication of where you are weakest. Most of us have a dominant side. The use of kettlebells can help balance out the differences between our more dominant side and less dominant side. It is important to improve muscle balance to reduce the risk of injury during normal day-to-day activities as well as during sport and exercise.

Simplicity - The minimalist concept of kettlebells keeps your workout routine simple. Because kettlebells can provide a total body workout, you don't need multiple pieces of equipment to achieve your goals. Multiple pieces of equipment can be overwhelming, intimidating, and expensive. You can simplify your workout routine by using one piece of equipment. People often make the mistake of thinking they have to have multiple pieces of equipment for their workouts to be effective. Nothing could be further from the truth. Workout routines using kettlebells can be simple and effective and help you achieve your desired results at a much faster rate. Most exercises are easy to learn and with the click of a mouse, you can find endless instructional videos to help ensure you are performing exercises correctly.

Whether your overall goal is weight loss, strength gain, speed, power, or overall fitness, kettlebells are an effective solution for your workout routine. They are functional, simple to use, and a great way to get the most out of your home workouts. If you are limited on space or money, you can create your own personal garage gym with one simple piece of equipment. For individuals who are new to working out, kettlebells are an excellent way for you to achieve your overall goals while working out at home.

How To

AMRAP Workouts: These workouts are designed to be repeated for the designated amount of time. To increase intensity, track and record how many rounds you can complete in the given time. Try to beat your score the next time you complete the workout.

Rounds For Time Workouts: These workouts are designed to be repeated for the given number of rounds. To increase intensity, record how long it takes you to complete the workout. Try to beat your time the next time you complete the workout.

Ladder Workouts: These workouts are designed to be completed in a ladder, meaning you add one more exercise every round. For example, your first round will be the first exercise. Your second round will be the second and first exercises. Your third round will be the third, second, and first exercises, and so on. Your final round will consist of all exercises. To increase intensity, record how long it takes you to complete the workout. Try to beat your time the next time you complete the workout.

Tabata Workouts: Tabata workouts consist of 20 seconds of the given exercise followed by 10 seconds of rest. Complete the given rounds of each exercise before moving on to the next one. For example, complete 8 rounds of tabata squats (20 seconds on / 10 seconds off) before moving on to tabata pushups.

Every Minute on the Minute Workouts (EMOM): These workouts are designed to be repeated every minute, on the minute, for the given number of minutes. After completing the reps, you have the remainder of the minute to rest.

Even/Odd Minute EMOM: These workouts are designed to be repeated every minute, on the minute, for the given number of minutes. In this case, however, all reps of the first exercise are to be completed in the first minute and all reps of the second exercise are to be completed the next minute. After completing the reps, you have the remainder of each minute to rest.

Deck of Cards: For these workouts you will need a deck of cards. Each suit will have an exercise assigned to it. The number on the card represents the number of reps to be performed for the corresponding exercise. Face cards equal 10 reps. A's equal 11 reps.

Scaling and Intensity

<u>**Scaling Workouts**</u>

Decrease Weight. Try using a lighter kettlebell and completing the workout with the recommended reps.

Decrease Reps. Try a lower number of reps than recommended in order to complete the workouts. For example, do 3 or 5 pull ups per round if you are unable to do 10.

Use Aid. Use a band to aid with pull ups if you can't do strict pull ups. Do pistol squats to a box or chair. Etc…

Modify Exercise. Modify an exercise if needed. For example, try air squats instead of goblet squats or sit ups instead of v ups.

<u>**Increase Intensity:**</u>

Increase Weight.

Minimize Rest.

Use a timer. Always try to get as much work done as possible in the given time.

Log each workout. Log your total rounds, time, reps, etc. Try to beat that total next time you attempt the workout.

AMRAPs

<u>18 Minutes of...</u>
10 KB High Pulls
10 KB Goblet Squats
10 Pull Ups

<u>20 Minutes of...</u>
10 KB Ballistic Rows
10 Burpees
10 Pull Ups
10 KB Bottoms Up Presses

<u>15 Minutes of...</u>
10 Burpees
20 KB Swings

<u>18 Minutes of...</u>
10 KB High Pulls
10 Push Ups
10 Sit Ups

<u>20 Minutes of...</u>
10 KB Cleans (each side)
5 KB Turkish Get Ups (each side)

<u>20 Minutes of...</u>
5 Pull Ups
10 KB Ballistic Rows
15 Push Ups

20 Minutes of…
12 KB Goblet Squats
12 Burpees
12 Sit Ups

20 Minutes of…
10 KB Single Leg Deadlifts (each side)
10 KB Bottoms Up Presses (each side)
100 Jump Rope

18 Minutes of…
10 KB Snatches (each side)
10 Burpees

20 Minutes of…
20 Alternating Single Arm KB Swings
20 Push Ups
250m Row

15 Minutes of…
20 Alternating KB Snatches
10 Pull Ups

18 Minutes of…
12 KB Squat Cleans
12 Burpees

20 Minutes of…
10 KB Single Arm Squat Cleans (each side)
10 Box Jumps
10 Pull Ups

<u>18 Minutes of</u>
5 Pull Ups
10 KB Ballistic Rows
15 Sit Ups

<u>20 Minutes of…</u>
10 KB High Pulls
10 Box Jumps
10 Burpees

<u>20 Minutes of…</u>
5 Turkish Get Ups (each side)
20 Russian Twists

<u>20 Minutes of…</u>
20 KB Alternating Side Lunges
20 Push Ups
20 Sit Ups

<u>20 Minutes of…</u>
400m Run
40 KB Swings
40 Sit Ups

<u>18 Minutes of…</u>
12 KB Swings
12 Box Jumps
12 Push Ups

<u>20 Minutes of…</u>
5 Pull Ups
10 KB Snatches
15 Jump Squats

20 Minutes of...

10 KB Goblet Squats

20 Alternating KB Snatches

30 Calorie Row

20 Minutes of...

10 Pull Ups

20 KB Swings

30 Walking Lunges

20 Minutes of...

20 Alternating Single Arm KB Swings

20 Walking Lunges

20 Calorie Row

18 Minutes of...

5 Single Arm KB Squat Cleans (each side)

10 Pull Ups

20 Minutes of...

10 KB High Pulls

10 KB Goblet Squats

100m KB Farmers Carry

20 Minutes of...

10 KB Snatches (each side)

10 KB Goblet Squats

10 KB Halos

20 Minutes of...

5 Box Jumps

10 KB Swings

15 Push Ups

ROUNDS FOR TIME

8 Rounds
5 KB Squat Cleans Left Side
5 Pull Ups
5 KB Squat Cleans Right Side
5 Pull Ups

5 Rounds
12 KB Goblet Squats
12 Burpees
12 Sit Ups

10 Rounds
5 Single Arm KB Squat Cleans (each side)
10 Burpees

5 Rounds
20 Alternating KB Step Back Lunges
20 Push Ups

5 Rounds
10 KB Snatches (each side)
10 Pull Ups

5 Rounds
10 KB High Pulls
10 Pull Ups
10 KB Goblet Squats
10 Burpees
10 KB Swings
100 Jump Rope

3 Rounds
10 Burpees
20 Pull Ups
30 Push Ups
40 KB Ballistic Rows
50 Alternating KB Snatches

3 Rounds
50 Calorie Row
40 KB Swings
30 Burpees
20 KB High Pulls
10 Pull Ups

5 Rounds
5 Single Arm KB Overhead Squats (each side)
5 KB Turkish Get Ups (each side)

5 Rounds
5 KB Snatches (each side)
5 KB Single Arm Squat Cleans (each side)
5 KB Turkish Get Ups (each side)

5 Rounds
10 KB Swings
10 Box Jumps
10 Burpees

5 Rounds
10 KB Halos
10 KB Side Bends
10 KB Russian Twists
100m KB Farmers Carry

5 Rounds

5 KB Squat Clean and Presses (each side)
10 Pull Ups
10 Box Jumps

6 Rounds

12 KB Goblet Squats
12 T Push Ups

5 Rounds

20 KB Swings
20 Push Ups
20 Calorie Row

2 Rounds

10 Burpees
20 KB High Pulls
30 KB Goblet Squats
40 Push Ups
50 KB Swings
40 Push Ups
30 KB Goblet Squats
20 KB High Pulls
10 Burpees

5 Rounds

10 KB High Pulls
10 KB Halos
10 Burpees

5 Rounds

10 KB Halos
10 Pull Ups
100 Flutter Kicks

6 Rounds

12 Goblet Squats
12 Box Jumps
12 Push Ups

4 Rounds

10 Pull Ups
20 KB High Pulls

5 Rounds

10 KB Goblet Squats
20 KB Ballistic Rows
30 Mountain Climbers

10 Rounds

5 Box Jumps
10 KB High Pulls
15 Push Ups

5 Rounds

5 Turkish Get Ups Right
5 Pull Ups
5 Turkish Get Ups Left
5 Pull Ups

5 Rounds

25 KB Goblet Squats
50m KB Farmer Carry Left
25 Sit Ups
50m Farmer Carry Right

<u>5 Rounds</u>
10 Pull Ups
20 KB Ballistic Rows
30 Sit Ups

<u>1 Round</u>
Half Mile Run
50 Pull Ups
50 Push Ups
50 KB Goblet Squats
50 KB Swings
Half Mile Run

<u>10,0,8,7,6,5,4,3,2,1 Reps of…</u>
KB Thrusters
Burpees

<u>10,9,8,7,6,5,4,3,2,1 Reps of…</u>
KB Single Arm Squat Cleans (each side)
Burpees

<u>10,9,8,7,6,5,4,3,2,1 Reps of…</u>
KB Snatches (each side)
Pull Ups

<u>10,9,8,7,6,5,4,3,2,1 Reps of…</u>
KB Snatches (each side)
Pistol Squats (each leg)

<u>10,9,8,7,6,5,4,3,2,1 Reps of…</u>
KB Thrusters
Pull Ups

10,9,8,7,6,5,4,3,2,1 Reps of...
KB Single Leg Deadlifts (each leg)
KB Bottoms Up Presses (each arm)
Pull Ups

10,9,8,7,6,5,4,3,2,1 Reps of...
KB Single Leg Deadlifts (each leg)
KB Bottoms Up Presses (each arm)
Burpees

10,9,8,7,6,5,4,3,2,1 Reps of...
KB Snatches (each side)
Box Jumps

50,40,30,20,10 Reps of...
KB Swings
Push Ups

50,40,30,20,10 Reps of...
Alternating KB Snatches
Alternating KB Lunges

50,40,30,20,10 Reps of...
KB Squat Cleans
Push Ups

50,40,30,20,10 Reps of...
KB Ballistic Rows
Sit Ups

EMOM WORKOUTS

EMOM for 10 Minutes
7 KB High Pulls
7 Burpees

EMOM for 10 Minutes
5 Box Jumps
15 KB Swings

EMOM for 8 Minutes
10 KB High Pulls
10 KB Goblet Squats
10 Push Ups

EMOM for 10 Minutes
5 Pull Ups
15 KB Swings

EMOM for 12 Minutes
10 KB High Pulls
10 Jump Squats
10 Jump Lunges

EMOM for 10 Minutes
10 KB Goblet Squats
10 KB Ballistic Rows

EMOM for 20 Minutes
5 Pull Ups
10 KB Halos
10 Sit Ups

EMOM for 10 Minutes
Even Minutes: 20 Alternating KB Snatches
Odd Minutes: 10 Pull Ups

EMOM for 12 Minutes
Even Minutes: 20 Alternating KB Lunges
Odd Minutes: 20 Up Down Planks

EMOM for 20 Minutes
Even Minutes: 5 KB Squat Cleans (each side)
Odd Minutes: 10 Box Jumps

EMOM for 12 Minutes
Even Minutes: 5 Turkish Get Ups Left Side
Odd Minutes: 5 Turkish Get Ups Right Side

EMOM for 12 Minutes
Even Minutes: 10 Box Jumps
Odd Minutes: 20 KB Goblet Squats

EMOM for 18 Minutes
Even Minutes: 10 KB Squat Cleans
Odd Minutes: 10 Burpees

EMOM for 12 Minutes
Even Minutes: 20 Alternating KB Lunges
Odd Minutes: 10 Burpees

LADDER WORKOUTS

Ladder
5 Burpees
10 KB Halos
15 KB Goblet Squats
20 Jump Lunges
25 Sit Ups
30 Mountain Climbers

Ladder
5 Pull Ups
10 Burpees
15 KB Single Leg Deadlifts
20 KB High Pulls
25 Mountain Climbers
30 V-Ups

Ladder
5 Pull Ups
10 KB Snatches (each side)
15 Up/Down Planks
20 KB Swings
25 Squats
30 Burpees

Ladder
5 Burpees
10 Diamond Push Ups
15 KB Goblet Squats
20 Reverse KB Lunges
25 KB Swings
30 Straight Leg Sit Ups

Ladder
10 Box Jumps
20 Straight Leg Sit Ups
30 KB High Pulls
40 Push Ups

Ladder
10 Burpees
20 KB Goblet Squats
30 Walking KB Lunges
40 Toe Touches

INTERVAL WORKOUTS

3 Rounds
1 Minute of Burpees
1 Minute of Alternating KB Swings
1 Minute of Push Ups
1 Minute of Sit Ups
1 Minute of Plank
1 Minute Rest

3 Rounds
1 Minute of KB Ballistic Rows
1 Minute of Squats
1 Minute of KB Halos
1 Minute of Alternating Lunges
1 Minute of Burpees
1 Minute Rest

3 Rounds
1 Minute of Rower
1 Minute of Box Jumps
1 Minute of Alternating Lunges
1 Minute of Alternating KB Snatches
1 Minute of Sit Ups
1 Minute Rest

3 Rounds
1 Minute of Burpees
1 Minute of KB Goblet Squats
1 Minute of Up Down Planks
1 Minute of KB High Pulls
1 Minute of Rower
1 Minute Rest

3 Rounds

1 Minute of Burpees
1 Minute of Goblet Squats
1 Minute of KB Ballistic Rows
1 Minute Assault Bike
1 Minute Plank
1 Minute Rest

Tabata

KB Swings
Box Jumps
KB Halos
Burpees

Tabata

KB High Pulls
Burpees
KB Ballistic Rows
Sit Ups

Tabata

Jump Squats
KB Halos
Jump Lunges
KB Ballistic Rows

Tabata

Row for Calories
Goblet Squats
Alternating Lunges
Russian Twists

Tabata

Burpees
KB Swings
Push Ups
Sit Ups

DECK OF CARDS

Cards
Hearts: KB Goblet Squats
Diamonds: Jump Squats
Spades: Alternating KB Lunges
Clubs: Jump Lunges

Cards
Hearts: KB Squat Cleans
Diamonds: KB Halos
Spades: Box Jumps
Clubs: Sit Ups

Cards
Hearts: KB Ballistic Rows
Diamonds: KB Halos
Spades: Push Ups
Clubs: Sit Ups

Cards
Hearts: Left Leg Single Leg KB Deadlifts
Diamonds: Right Leg Single Leg KB Deadlifts
Spades: Push Ups
Clubs: Pull Ups

Cards
Hearts: Left Arm KB Bottoms Up Press
Diamonds: Right Arm KB Bottoms Up Press
Spades: Pull Ups
Clubs: Sit Ups

Cards

Hearts: KB Swings
Diamonds: KB Goblet Squats
Spades: KB Ballistic Rows
Clubs: Push Ups